Seeing Beyond the Wrinkles

Study Guide for Personal Reflection and Spiritual Growth

A companion to
Seeing Beyond the Wrinkles, 2nd edition
ISBN: 1-882349-06-7 • LC: 98-75225

Charles Tindell

Studio 4 Productions
Northridge, California

SEEING BEYOND THE WRINKLES
Study Guide for Personal Reflection
and Spiritual Growth

© 1999 by Studio 4 Productions
All rights reserved
First Printing 1999

Studio 4 Productions
P.O. Box 280400
Northridge, CA 91328-0400
U.S.A.

ISBN: 1-882349-06-7

Library of Congress Catalog Card Number: 98-75225

Editor: Joel Leach
Book Design: Carey Christensen
Cover Design: Robert Aulicino

Scripture quotations from:
HOLY BIBLE, New International Version (NIV)
©1973,1978,1984, International Bible Society
Used by permission of Zondervan Publishing House.

"Do not cast me away when I am old;
do not forsake me when my strength is gone."

Psalm 71:9 (NIV)

Contents

Stories are grouped thematically
and appear in the same order as in the text
Seeing Beyond the Wrinkles,
Stories of Ageless Courage, Humor, and Faith

Preface

The questions in this study guide are meant to encourage discussion and will hopefully raise other questions. Adapt the questions for your situation. Suggested ways that this study guide, along with *Seeing Beyond the Wrinkles*, may be used are:

- Small group study.
- Retreats.
- Personal devotion booklet.
- A training resource for those who visit the elderly as part of their ministry within their communities of faith, for example, Stephen Ministry, Befrienders, etc.
- Sunday school.
- Adult education.
- A catalyst for conversation and discussion while visiting someone in a nursing home or retirement center.
- For personal reflection upon one's own journey through life, especially as one faces their own aging process.
- To reflect upon the aging process of a relative or friend, and perhaps to be personally challenged to look upon older persons in a different light (to see beyond the wrinkles).

There are *no answers* in the back of the book because individuals will become personally involved as they deal with the questions from where they are at in their life experiences and journey of faith. You are encouraged to write your answers in a notebook or a journal.

There is a reflection section corresponding to each theme. It begins with a biblical quote (NIV) followed by some introductory remarks, and then questions to reflect upon. It ends with a prayer.

Many of the sections have biblical verses and stories from which to refer. All sections have a spiritual foundation upon which it stands and will challenge you to grow in your faith.

1

Stereotypes

"He replied, 'The man they call Jesus made some mud and put it on my eyes. He told me to go to Siloam and wash. So I went and washed, and then I could see.'"

John 9:11 (NIV)

Jesus was always talking about those who have eyes but do not see. What was true then is no less true today. We live in a world where, because of prejudices and stereotypes, we are blind to who people really are. There are those who cannot see beyond the color of another's skin, ethnic background, religious identity, or wrinkles.

The Gospel is always meant to open our eyes. Our Lord told us that the truth shall make us free. Only when we see people for who they are can we ourselves truly be free.

1. Name some groups of people who are cast in prejudicial stereotypes.
    a. In what ways are they viewed in a negative manner?
    b. Can being stereotyped *imprison* people? In what ways?
    c. Can we ourselves be imprisoned by the stereotypes we have of others? How?
2. What kind of stereotypes do people generally have of the elderly?
    a. How do their stereotypes affect the way they interact with them?
    b. How are the stereotypes reinforced by television and movies?
    c. In what ways might we change these stereotypes?
3. Do you recall the first time you ever visited someone in a nursing home? What were your feelings about it before and after the visit?

4. What is your perception of what nursing homes were like 20 years ago? Have they changed over the years? If so, in what ways? In what ways have they remained the same?
5. Think of an elderly friend or relative. Does that person fit the stereotypical image of the elderly? What is especially unique about him/her that helps shatter that image?
6. Have you ever experienced others being "blind" to where you are in your own aging process?
    a. What were the circumstances?
    b. How did that blindness make you feel?
7. How would you feel if it were necessary for you to spend your last days as a nursing home resident?
    a. What would you like to tell people (staff, family, members of your faith community) about how you would like to be treated if that should happen?
    b. What would be your concerns and/or fears if it should happen?
8. When we think of playfulness and creative use of imagination, we so often first think of children. Why is it so hard to think of the elderly in such a way?
    a. What are the differences between being *childish* and *child-like?*
    b. When was the last time you were child-like, and what were the circumstances?
9. In the story about *Violet,* she talked about the sensation of standing apart from oneself in order to better view oneself, If you did that now, who would you see?

Prayer
   Help us to be sensitive to the blind spots we have in our dealings with others and especially with the elderly. Forgive us when we judge others in ways that we ourselves would not like to be judged. Anoint our eyes with the cleansing power of the clay so that we might see all people for who they are. Amen.

2

Uniqueness

"When I consider your heavens, the work of your fingers, the moon and the stars, which you have set in place, what is man that you are mindful of him, the son of man that you care for him?"

Psalm 8:3-4 (NIV)

The Scriptures repeatedly point out the uniqueness of the individual within the scheme of God's creation. When Jesus tells us not to conform to the ways of the world but be transformed, he is sharing with us a spiritual truth which affirms the worth of each person as he or she is transformed by the power of the Gospel. We have worth as creations of God's love and we can only fully understand that truth once we undergo transformation and no longer try to establish our value based on the standards of the world in which we live.

1. List some things which give individuals a sense of self-worth. Which of these things would apply to you? Discuss the importance of having a sense of self-worth.
2. Of those listed in question 1, which would apply to a 92-two-year-old stroke victim who spends most of his time sitting in a wheelchair? If none of them would apply, what could you say to this man that would affirm his sense of worth?
3. In what ways does our society contribute to the feelings of worthlessness among the elderly?
4. Have you ever felt like a "dust speck?" If so, under what circumstances? (For example, you might feel like a cog in the wheel where you work, or just one of the "residents" in a nursing home.)

5. If scientists were to discover that the earth is the only place in the universe that has life forms, would that make you feel more like a dust speck? Why, or why not?
6. How are individuals or groups valued within society? Can you think of examples of those who are valued mainly for their:
   a. material possessions
   b. power or influence
   c. youth
   d. productivity
7. Have you ever known a person of whom it was said, "They broke the mold when he/she was made"? What was so special about that person?
   a. Do you believe that they broke the mold when *you* were made?
   b. Why did you answer 7a the way you did?
8. Share the unique qualities of an older person whom you know or have known.
9. What groups of people in society are being given the message that they are "valueless?"
   a. Do you feel as though you are in one of those groups? If so, which one(s)?
   b. What would help to make you feel that you have value?
10. How can your community of faith place value on its elderly?
11. According to your spiritual beliefs, what place do you have within creation?
12. At your Service of Remembrance (see Opal's story), what would you like to be shared as a way of letting others know that you were unique?

Prayer
Grant us a clear vision so that we might see the value of each individual, beginning with ourselves. We pray also for spiritual insight so that we might discern how each individual, regardless of their situation or condition, is a valued member of our faith community. Amen.

3

Role Models

"But a Samaritan, as he traveled, came where the man was; and when he saw him, he took pity on him. He went to him and bandaged his wounds, pouring on oil and wine. Then he put the man on his own donkey, took him to an inn and took care of him."

Luke 10:33-34 (NIV)

Those who live in a long term care facility are attended to by a host of professional caregivers including nurses, therapists, social workers, dietitians, and those who help residents handle their finances. Caregivers also include housekeepers, volunteers, those engaged in providing activities, etc. All of these persons and more comprise a holistic approach to providing total care to the residents. Staff members serve as role models for caregiving, but then, so do the residents themselves also serve as role models for caregiving.

One of the benefits of working in a nursing home is that we who are caregivers receive as much care from the residents as we attempt to give. Professional caregivers soon discover that the elderly can not only teach them about how life was back in the "good old days" but also about life itself and what it means to care for others. If you are looking for role models, you only need to visit a nursing home.

1. Can you identify situations or circumstances in which you consider yourself to be a caregiver?
2. Have you ever attempted to cheer up someone whom you felt was in need, only to be cheered up yourself by that person's faith and positive attitude toward life? If so, who?
   a. What were the circumstances?

    b. How did you feel afterwards? Why do you think you felt that way?

3. Discuss the following: *There are always two needs whenever a visit is made to a resident in a nursing home (or someone in the hospital): the needs of the person making the visit and the needs of the person being visited.* Why is it important to understand the distinction between the two?

4. Name three attributes (more if possible) which you consider to be important for a person to have in order to be a good caregiver.

5. Which of those attributes listed in question 4 do you feel you have?

    a. Which do you feel need improvement?

    b. How might you improve them?

6. Read John 21:15-17, and reflect upon what those verses say about caregiving.

7. Who in society and the world would you consider to be the spiritual heroes and/or role models of today?

8. From your family or circle of friends, whom would you select as your spiritual hero and/or role model?

    a. Why did you select that particular person?

    b. What qualities do you admire most in that person?

9. Care giving also means self-care. In what ways do you take care of yourself?

    a. Are you satisfied with your self-care? Why or why not?

    b. In what ways could you improve on your self-care?

11. In what ways did Jesus do self-care?

12. Discuss what role modeling for your faith would mean.

Prayer

    Thank you for the caregivers in our lives, especially those who are teaching us through role modeling what it means to care for others. Grant us the wisdom to follow in their footsteps. Amen.

4

Joyfulness

"This is the day the Lord has made; let us rejoice and be glad in it."

Psalm 118:24 (NIV)

The Psalmist who penned the above words no doubt had days of struggle and pain just as the rest of us do. He was not, however, trying to gloss over such days as if to imply the person of faith simply puts on "rose-colored" glasses in difficult times through which to view the world. Rather, the verse is a proclamation to live by faith on a daily basis. And in spite of whatever the day may bring, we can still be joyful in the knowledge that the Lord will be with us. With that foundational faith to stand upon, we then can rejoice in each day.

1. On a scale of 1 to 10, with 10 being the highest, rate your sense of humor. Are you satisfied with your rating? Why or why not?
2. Why do you think it is good to have a sense of humor?
   a. From what side of the family did you inherit your sense of humor?
   b. When was the last time you had a good, cleansing laugh? What were the circumstances?
3. What constitutes good, healthy humor? Give examples. What is bad, unhealthy humor? Explain.
4. Why was Pearl's story called a story of triumph?
5. Why do you think people do not often think of the elderly as having a sense of humor?
   a. Do you know an older person who is a joy to be around, and who laughs easily? Describe that person's kind of joy.
   b. Share a memory of your parents or grandparents laughing. What was the occasion?

6. Reflect upon these words: "A cheerful heart is good medicine, but a crushed spirit dries up the bones." Proverbs 17:22 (NIV)
   a. Can a person confined to a wheelchair have a "cheerful heart?"
   b. Can a young person have "dried up bones?" Give examples.
   c. How can youth and older people help each other to rejoice?
7. Keeping Anabel's story in mind, have you ever had an older person invite you to laugh *with* them about the difficulties of growing old?
   a. Who? What were the circumstances?
   b. Did the experience change your feelings or attitude about older people in any way? If so, how?
8. List some concrete things you or your community of faith could do to provide "cheerful medicine" to those living in a nursing home:
9. Give examples of how one can rejoice in one's faith.
10. Do you think Jesus had a sense of humor? Why or why not?
11. What is the most joyful part of worship for you? Why? How do you express your joyfulness of faith in everyday life?
12. Keeping Sherman's story in mind, give examples of times when dancing is part of the celebration of events in one's life.
13. What would you think Sherman might say to King David? (see II Samuel 6:14-15)

Prayer

Open our ears to your joyful laughter, O Lord, and have us see each day as a precious gift in which we can rejoice. Fill us with such a spirit of sacred joyfulness that it overflows into all that we do or say. Amen.

9

5

Wisdom

"...for wisdom is more precious than rubies, and nothing you desire can compare with her."

Proverbs 8:11 (NIV)

While Vivienne's story speaks to the ever changing nature of life, Bill's story reminds us not to rush getting old, while enjoying life while we can. Amen Corner invites us to look at the world of the elderly from their particular corner. And Ben's story reminds us how God works in mysterious ways.

The quote from Proverbs reminds us that the most valuable thing we can have as we face life is wisdom. Each of the individuals whose stories make up this section reflect the wisdom of the ages.

1. How has your life changed in the past ten years?
   a. What changes were under your control?
   b. Which were not?
2. How did the changes in question 1 affect your walk of faith?
3. What wisdom was passed down to help you deal with the changes in life?
   a. From whom did the wisdom come?
   b. What wisdom would you like to pass on to the next generation?
4. Where is your *Amen Corner*—the place from which you can observe the world go by? What have you learned about yourself and the world from that spot?
5. It has been said that there is a moment of truth for all of us when we realize that we actually are aging.
   a. When, if ever, was that moment for you?
   b. What has been, or will be, the most difficult birthday for you? Why?

   c. What has been the most difficult change for you in recent years? Why?

6. In reference to Vivienne's story, what do you think her mother meant about "being patient with life?" Do you think you are patient with life? Explain.

7. What are some of the changeless attributes of God?
   a. Which of those have been the most reassuring for you?
   b. Are there any attributes that you have seen in a new light over the years? If so, in what way?

8. In what area of your life do you need to pray for wisdom? Why that particular area?

9. Discuss the difference between *wisdom* and *knowledge*. Can you have the *knowledge* of God while lacking spiritual wisdom? Explain.

10. Looking back through the years, do you feel as though your faith has increased, remained the same, or decreased? Explain.
   a. What views of God have changed within our society?
   b. What views of God have remained constant?

11. Ben says in his story that God works in mysterious ways. Has God ever worked in mysterious ways within your life? If so, when? Under what circumstances? What did you learn from those experiences?

12. In Bill's story, he tells us not to rush getting old. What do you think he means by that?

Prayer

As we deal with the ever-changing nature of this life, grant us wisdom to rely and trust in the changeless truths of the Kingdom of God. We ask for wisdom and insight as we ponder all the ways you speak to us of spiritual truths. Guide us to proclaim them from generation to generation. We pray this in the name of Jesus, the Alpha and the Omega. Amen.

6

Love

"And now these three remain: faith, hope and love. But the greatest of these is love."

I Corinthians 13:13 (NIV)

There are three main words used to convey the notion of love in New Testament Greek. The first one is *eros*, which is a longing, a desire or a physical attraction two individuals may have for one another. The second is *phileo* which denotes the love that friends or relatives have for one another. The third is *agape*. *Agape* is the kind of love mentioned in the verse found in the 13th chapter of Corinthians. It refers to the Christ-like love one is to demonstrate toward others; it is a way of life based on God's love.

1. Thinking in particular of your parents and grandparents, share examples of each of the three kinds of love that you witnessed.
   a. Eros
   b. Phileo
   c. Agape
2. What lessons about love did you learn from your parents and grandparents?
3. Read I Corinthians 13. Share examples of how one could show agape love among:
   a. Your family
   b. Your friends
   c. Co-workers
   d. Your faith community
   e. Nursing home residents
4. Discuss how agape can influence eros and phileo.
5. Do you think agape is something we do naturally or is it something one must learn? Explain and discuss.

6. Share examples of times when you believe you were on the receiving end of agape.
7. Read John 3:16 and reflect upon the following:
    a. Is understanding God's love for us the same as understanding the *depth* of God's feeling of love?
    b. How might we begin to understand God's feeling of love through our relationships? (Consider, for example, sacrifices parents make for their children; also consider watching someone whom we love make wrongful life decisions.)
8. How do you see the following fitting in with Isabelle's closing remark in her story:
    a. I Corinthians 13:13
    b. Leviticus 19:18
    c. John 15:17
    d. I John 4:19
9. Do you know of people who are abiding in God's love? If so, who?
    a. Share their stories.
    b. What have you personally learned from their lives?
10. According to John 15:9, Jesus tells us to "remain in my love." What do you think Jesus means by that and how might it affect our everyday lives?
11. While keeping the story *Huddling* in mind, discuss the following: Life is a series of hellos and good-byes. The good-byes are never easy. The only way to live life without experiencing the pain of separation when someone dies, is to go through life without investing your love in others. God has given us another option: that is to love.
    a. Which option have you chosen and why? Is it easy to choose that option? Explain.
    b. Jesus tells us to love our enemies. How can you love the enemies in your life?
12. What does the concept of God's unconditional love mean to you? Have you experienced it? If so, in what ways?

Prayer

Thank you for your love which sustains us day-by-day. Help us to demonstrate that love in all our relationships. Grant us the wisdom to understand that we may get too old for a number of things but we are never too old to love. Amen.

7

Fortitude

"My soul is weary with sorrow; strengthen me according to your word."

Psalm 119:28 (NIV)

Having a long life is a blessing, but it can often be a mixed blessing. On the one hand, by living to be 80 or 90, we outlive most of our friends and unfortunately, sometimes, even our children. On the other hand, the elderly also have to cope with physical disabilities that so often come with aging. The latter years of one's life can be the most challenging physically, emotionally, mentally, and spiritually. It is during these years that one's fortitude is really tested.

1. Do you know older people who have outlived one or more of their children?
   a. Who were they? Share those stories.
   b. How did they cope? What helped them the most?
   c. Did they draw upon the resources of their faith? If so, was that helpful?
   d. What, if any, spiritual advice did they offer regarding their experience?
   e. What spiritual advice could you share if someone sought your advice?
2. Consider Mary's feelings about losing her 33-year-old son, Jesus. Try to imagine her emotional state as she watched him suffer and die on a cross: What kind of emotions would you be feeling if you were there?
3. With regard to older people you know, what kind of inner strengths did they exhibit as they coped with life?

4. If you knew you would have to move into a nursing home in the near future:
   a. What would be the most difficult part of the experience for you? Why?
   b. In what ways could you draw upon your faith to help make the transition easier for you?
5. Consider being 85-years-old and having to share a nursing home room with another person. Which qualities of the Spirit (See Galatians 5:22-23) would you need. Why those?
6. List 5 every-day things that would be affected if you had a stroke and one side of your body was paralyzed.
   a. How would you feel about these things?
   b. Which things would be most difficult for you to do?
   c. From where would you draw the strength necessary to help you cope?
7. Having reflected upon all the things that can happen when one grows older, read the words of Jesus in Matthew 6:25-34, and reflect upon what they mean as you look ahead at the coming years.
8. In the story, *Soulmates*, Mildred said that, through faith, she could learn from her pain.
   a. What do you think she meant?
   b. Have you had opportunities to learn from your pain? Give some examples and tell what you learned.
9. Do you think God causes pain and suffering in order to test or punish us? Explain.
10. On a scale of 1 to 10, with 10 being the highest, how would you rate your spiritual fortitude? Why did you rate yourself as you did?

Prayer

As you have been with us in the past, O Lord, remind us that you will be with us in the future. Grant us the wisdom to place our trust in you, knowing that we do not make the journey alone. Strengthen us with the knowledge that you are always with us. Amen.

Friendship

"I hope to see you soon, and we will talk face to face. Peace to you. The friends here send their greetings. Greet the friends there by name."

3 John 1:14 (NIV)

In writing to Gaius, a prominent Christian, the Apostle John commends him for his hospitality. John recognizes the importance of friendship and closes his letter by asking Gaius to greet his friends by name, for John hopes to see them soon.

Friendship is important and it truly is one of the blessings of God. As the stories in this section showed, friendship may come to us in many different ways, even through a teddy bear or a puppet by the name of August. However way it comes, it is good to have someone we can call a friend. The Bible reminds us that Jesus also wants to be our friend.

1. How would you define friendship? What are the characteristics of a good friend?
2. Name some people with whom you have been friends for a long time.
   a. How did those friendships begin?
   b. Why are these friendships important to you?
3. Have there been times in your life when you needed help from a friend? Give examples.
   a. How did you feel about receiving help?
   b. Was it hard for you to ask for help? If so, why do you think that was the case?
4. Have you experienced bonding with another person through:
   a. Sharing a hardship? What was it? In what ways did it bond you together?
   b. Crying or sharing a deep sorrow? With whom? Explain the circumstances.

c. Laughter or joy? With whom? Explain the circumstances.

d. Praying together or sharing some other deep spiritual experience? With whom? Explain the circumstances?

5. We celebrate birthdays and wedding anniversaries. Can you think of ways in which a friendship might be celebrated? How do you presently celebrate your friendships?

6. In the stories we read about how a teddy bear and a puppet by the name of August could be a friend.

   a. Did you have a favorite stuffed animal as a child?

   b. What do you remember about it? Did it have a name?

   c. Can you get in touch with any feelings attached to your stuffed animal? If so, what are they?

   d. Discuss how such inanimate objects can be "friends."

7. In terms of friendships and/or relationships, reflect upon the following passages:

   a. Matthew 11:19

   b. Proverbs 17:17

   c. James 4:4-5

   d. Proverbs 19:6

   e. Matthew 5:25

   f. John 15:14-17

8. Did you grow up with the concept of God as a friend? If so, explain.

9. God's friendship means that we can receive help from God. Reflect upon the following verses in terms of what kind of help is being offered:

   a. Psalm 46:1

   b. Romans 8:26

   c. Mark 9:24

   d. Philippians 1:19

10. What does the hymn, *What a Friend We Have in Jesus,* mean to you?

11. Some people refer to others as their "friends in Christ." What do you think they mean by that? Do you have such friends? If so, share the characteristics of such friendships.

Prayer

We thank you for friends, past and present. We pray for wisdom so that we might be a friend to others as you have been unto us. Amen.

Caring

"The next day we landed at Sidon; and Julius, in kindness to Paul, allowed him to go to his friends so they might provide for his needs."

Acts 27:3 (NIV)

As the Apostle Paul sailed for Rome while in custody, he was befriended by Julius, a Roman soldier. Out of kindness this centurion allowed Paul to be cared for by friends. Paul, in faith, knew God would provide and watch over him. Throughout Paul's ministry he constantly gave of himself to the care of others. Through this encounter, however, Paul was now experiencing what it meant to be a care *receiver*.

All of us provide care for others and that is certainly good. Caregiving fits into theology as one of the important elements of ministry. However, there comes a time when we, ourselves, need to be cared for and comforted. It is so much better when that care and comfort is done by those who know and love us.

1. List 4 characteristics of what you would expect to find in a community where its members truly care for one another.
    a.
    b.
    c.
    d.
2. In what ways do the following communities (of which you are a part) provide care for their members:
    a. Family
    b. Circle of friends
    c. Workplace
    d. Community of faith

3. Are there any ways in which the care shown in the communities of question 2 could be improved? Share your thoughts.
4. Share examples of caring for each other that you have witnessed between your parents or grandparents.
5. Do you think it is easier to be a caregiver or a care receiver? Explain.
6. If you had a family member or friend living in a nursing home, what could you suggest that he or she might do in order to show more caring for other residents and for the staff?
7. How does your faith community care for the elderly? Do you believe it could do more? If so, what?
8. Have you ever taken care of one who was elderly? Who was that? What were the circumstances?
   a. What kind of emotions did you have during the period you cared for that person?
   b. Did you learn any lessons about life from the person? If so, what?
9. The comment was made in the story, *Two Nurses*, that "it is a special privilege to be present at the moment of death."
   a. Would you like to be with your loved ones when they died? Why or why not?
   b. Would you like to have a family member or friend there when you die? Why or why not?
10. What would you expect from those who care for you in your last days?
    a. What would be important to you?
    b. What would not be important to you?
11. What do the following verses tell us about caring:
    a. I Corinthians 12:25-26
    b. John 10:1-18
    c. Luke 10:29-37
    d. I Peter 5:7

Prayer

We thank you for all those who have cared for us over the years (name them aloud or within your heart). Grant us the wisdom to continue to care for others we now name (name them aloud or within your heart). We ask that we might be shown ways in which we might touch the lives of others with the loving care you have shown us. Amen.

19

Storytellers

"He told them another parable..."

Matthew 13:31 (NIV)

The Bible has often been referred to as God's story of salvation. As one studies the different books within the Bible we get a picture of who God is and how we fit into the story of God's grace. Throughout the pages of Scripture there is the admonition to hear the story that is being unfolded so that we may share it with others. In sharing the story with others, we are also sharing the essence of who we are as the people of God and what is important to us in life.

Jesus often told parables (earthly stories with heavenly meaning) that pointed to various truths about the Kingdom of God. His parables appealed to all ages because they were drawn from the ordinary events of life.

1. Who are the storytellers within your family? Why are they important to your family?
   a. Share a story you have often heard at family gatherings.
   b. Why do you think the story in 1a is often told?
2. Share a story about yourself or a family member which tells something about your:
   a. Sense of humor
   b. Values
   c. Faith
3. If you wrote your autobiography, what title would you give it? Why would you choose that title?
4. Is anyone recording *your* family stories?
   a. If so, how are they doing it?
   b. To whom will these stories be passed on?

5. List some ways in which stories could be "recorded" to be passed on to the next generation (keep in mind today's technology).
6. Share any "faith stories" you have as you remember the following:
   a. A death in the family
   b. Family devotions or church attendance
   c. Family gathering for a holiday or birthday
   d. A family crisis
7. Discuss what being able to share stories might mean to an older person in terms of their:
   a. Dignity
   b. Self worth
   c. Standing within the family
8. Do you feel we live in a society in which older people are respected for their storytelling? Discuss.
9. Are there people you know who could be seen as *living history lessons?* Who?
   a. Why do you believe that is so?
   b. What history lessons have you learned from those people?
10. In what ways do the following stories help us understand the truths of the Kingdom of God:
    a. Matthew 25:1-13
    b. Luke 12:16-21
    c. Luke 16:1-9
    d. Matthew 18:21-35
11. Do you have a favorite Bible story? If so, share it. Why is that story your favorite?
12. List the many ways your community of faith shares the story of the Gospel.
13. In what ways could your faith community tap into the journey-of-faith stories that older people have to share?

Prayer
We thank you for the storytellers within our midst. Grant us the wisdom to take the time to listen to their stories for by so doing, our lives—as well as theirs—will be enriched. Encourage us also to share the story of your Kingdom with all of those with whom we come into contact. Help us to witness to the truths we have discovered with the story of the Gospel. Amen.

11

Listening

"Then a cloud appeared and enveloped them, and a voice came from the cloud: 'This is my Son, whom I love. Listen to him!'"

Mark 9:7 (NIV)

Listening. It seems like such a simple task, particularly when we consider the fact that it affects every segment of our lives. Counselors tell us that the inability or unwillingness to listen to one another causes one of the most significant problems a married couple experiences. Similarly, our spiritual lives falter because we so often fail to listen to God. Jesus is continually exhorting those who have ears to hear.

I wonder: Are the words found in Mark 9:7 a command, or could they be simply the pleading of a loving God who knows how much our lives would be enriched if only we would listen?

1. Make a list of characteristics you feel a good listener would have.
   a. How many of those characteristics do you think you have?
   b. How might you improve your listening skills?
2. Who are the "listeners" in your life? Why are they valuable to you?
3. When someone listens to you as you share a problem, do you also expect that person to fix it? Explain.
4. Make a list of people for whom you are "the listener."
   a. Does it take energy to listen? Explain.
   b. Do you ever feel too tired to listen? If so, what do you do when you feel that way?
5. How would you feel if you tried to tell something that was important to another person, only to realize that he or she was not listening?

6. In the event you know someone who suffers from short-term memory loss, do you think you will listen to that person differently after having read Esther's story?
   a. Share examples of elderly people you know who make it a point not to just sit around and complain.
   b. Have you ever felt you were *explaining* but yet were seen as *complaining*? Share that experience.
7. In thinking about what it means to listen, reflect upon the following:
   a. Matthew 11:15
   b. Proverbs 21:13
   c. John 8:47
   d. Psalms 61:1
8. Read Matthew 9:27-34 and reflect upon the following:
   a. Can we have 20/20 vision and yet, still be blind? Explain. Give examples.
   b. How can our sight be restored so that we might *listen* more to the Gospel?
   c. If having 20/20 vision meant seeing Jesus for who he is and having no questions or doubts, would your vision be 20/20? If not, what would it be? Why?
   d. What would it mean to be spiritually near-sighted (unable to see things that are far away)? Give examples.
   e. What would it mean to be spiritually far-sighted (unable to see things that are near)? Give examples.
9. In what ways to you listen to God?
10. Do you feel God always listens to your prayers? What about the prayers that seem to go unanswered? Does that mean God is not listening? Explain.

Prayer

Open our hearts so that we might listen to those who speak to us. Help us to hear those who are trying to explain where they are at in their journey of aging. Amen.

12

Memories

"Remember the days of old; consider the generations long past. Ask your father and he will tell you, your elders, and they will explain to you."

Deuteronomy 32:7 (NIV)

There are many kinds of treasures in the world. On one hand, there are those treasures which are of high monetary value; they are considered priceless. On the other hand, there are those which have very little monetary value, but which you also consider to be priceless. Memories may have no monetary value but they are certainly priceless treasures.

The elderly have a treasure chest full of memories waiting to be shared. When you visit them, take time to rummage through their treasure chests. If you do, you just may gain a better appreciation of your own treasures.

1. Share some treasures (toys or other possessions) you had as a child that even today, provide you with fond memories.
2. What are some of your earliest childhood memories (sounds, smells, favorite rooms, hiding places, etc.) of the home you grew up in?
3. What memories do you have of your parents or grandparents that have become part of your family's reminiscences from time to time?
   a. Why do you think these memories are important? What do they tell you about your family?
   b. Is there wisdom, or are there insights to life portrayed by these memories? If so, what are they?
4. What were some of the lessons about life taught to you as a child, by which you still try to live?
   a. Who (family, teachers, friends, etc.) taught those lessons to you?

b. Why are those lessons important to you?

5. In the story, *Orville*, there is mention of a "memory box." Name some items you would place in your memory box if you were ever to live in a nursing home. What do you think those items would say about you?

6. Share an experience you have had during which you felt the presence of God.
   a. With regard to your personal spiritual journey, is it important to remember this experience? If so, why?
   b. How does remembering that experience help you in your walk of faith at the present time?

7. Ecclesiastes 12:1 (NIV) tells us to "Remember your Creator in the days of your youth." As you reflect upon that thought, consider:
   a. Who helped shape your faith during your youth? In what ways were your faith shaped?
   b. Were these perceptions of God positive or negative? Elaborate.
   c. Have your ideas about God changed from your youth? If so, how?

8. What do the following scripture passages tell us about remembering and faith?
   a. Philippians 1:3
   b. Jeremiah 2:2
   c. Acts 20:35
   d. Revelation 3:3

9. Psalm 71:17-18 talks about lessons learned from God as a youth.
   a. What are your earliest recollections of *where* you were taught about God? (e.g. at home, Sunday School, Bible camp, etc.)
   b. Which of the lessons you learned about God during your youth have proven to be the most important to you through the years? Explain.

10. Reflecting upon Deuteronomy 32:7, consider the roles elders play in our lives.

11. Why do you think God wants us to remember the past?

Prayer

We remember with thanksgiving those who have helped guide our walk of faith through life, especially as they reminisce about their faith experiences. Amen.

13

Gifts

"We have different gifts, according to the grace given us...."

Romans 12:6 (NIV)

The Apostle Paul talks about the gifts we find within the community of the faithful. Certainly, there are the well-known gifts such as teaching and prophecy. Each of these gifts is seen as edifying the whole Body of Christ.

Though we continue to affirm the traditional gifts of the Spirit, there is also the need to recognize and celebrate gifts such as Agnes' quick wit. Her wit is a gift that brings smiles and warmth to those who are around her. Although confined to a wheelchair, she continues to be a bearer of gifts. As you reflect upon the questions below, think about intangible gifts such as a sense of humor, having compassion, a beautiful smile, or being a teller of tales.

1. Can you think of any gifts that are unique to the elderly which they could share with younger generations?
2. Name some gifts that are not affected by the passing of time.
3. Think about a grandparent or parent, and the gifts he or she shared.
   a. Name those gifts. Why were they important to you?
   b. Did age diminish those gifts? If so, in what way?
   c. Which of their gifts have become part of who you are now?
4. What gifts from your parents or grandparents would you like to take along with you in your later years?
5. Which of the gifts you received would you like to pass on to your family and friends? Are there certain gifts you

would like to see for certain people? (e.g., passing on your gift of the appreciation of music to a grandchild).

6. Does your community of faith have members who are in nursing homes or who are classified as "shut-ins?"
   a. Do you know what your community of faith is doing for those people? If so, what?
   b. Are there still other things that might be done? If so, give examples.
   c. Is there anything you would personally like to do for them?

7. Ask someone who knows you well to reflect upon your gifts. Next, share the gifts you see in that person's life.
   a. Which of your gifts are especially important to you as you face the aging process?
   b. Why are those gifts important?

8. Almeda talked about taking life "one day at a time."
   a. What does "taking one day at a time" mean to you?
   b. Is "taking one day at a time" something you try to practice? If so, what is the most difficult part of doing that? What would you tell someone who wanted to live by that philosophy?
   c. Read Matthew 6:34-35 and reflect upon what that concept means to you.

9. Would you like to live one hundred years? Why or why not?
   a. What would you fear the most about living to that age?
   b. What age would you like to live to? Why did you choose that age?

10. What are the three most important gifts God has given to you?

Prayer

Grant to us the ability to discern the many intangible gifts our elders have to share with us. Bless them for the many ways in which they benefit the whole community of faith. Amen.

14

Looking Back

"When Methuselah had lived 187 years, he became the father of Lamech. And after he became the father of Lamech, Methuselah lived 782 years and had other sons and daughters. Altogether, Methuselah lived 969 years, and then he died."

Genesis 5:25-27 (NIV)

The question as to whether Methuselah actually lived 969 years always comes up. Some argue that either years must have been measured differently in those times or that Methuselah's age referred to the years of his family dynasty and not to his individual age. Others believe that he *did* live that long. Regardless of which side one takes, the point the Bible is trying to make is that Methuselah lived to be a *very old man.* I wonder if Methuselah ever thought he would live to be as old as he did! Also, I wonder if, when he got to those later years, he grieved his youth.

People often associate grief and grieving only with the loss of a loved one through death. Grief, however, can be multi-dimensional and cumulative. It has been said that we are constantly in the process of grieving the loss of something or someone throughout our lives. Quite often, the elderly face a multitude of losses within a very short period of time.

1. *I Wonder if I Know* was written as a training exercise designed to help staff become more sensitive to the many losses residents go through as they enter nursing homes. There are at least 10 different kind of losses with which the woman in this scenario is dealing. Make a list of those losses and discuss them.

   a. Can you personally identify with any of those losses? In what way?

28

b. Which of those losses would be especially difficult for you? Explain.
2. Understanding that there are many different kinds of losses, share some you have experienced during the last 5 years:
    a. Which of those losses (other than the lost of loved ones) have been the most difficult?
    b. Have you ever grieved over things that you never thought you would miss? Explain and give examples.
3. Are there losses which occurred more than 5 years ago over which you still grieve? Name them.
    a. Have those losses become less painful with the passing of time? In what ways?
    b. What kind of impact have those losses had on your life?
    c. In what ways has your faith helped you cope with those losses?
4. What do the following scripture verses say to you about grieving?
    a. John 11:35
    b. I Thessalonians 4:13-14
    c. Romans 12:15
5. Reflect upon and discuss: Is it okay for people of faith to express grief even though they know their loved ones have gone "home to God?"
6. In Deuteronomy 34:18, God tells Moses that he will not live to enter the promised land. How do you think faith comes into play when one realizes that he or she may not realize their earthly dreams or desires?

Prayer
Comfort us in our grieving over the losses we have experienced and that we now name with our hearts. (Name them silently.) We offer thanks for the hope we share in the Good News and for a Savior who understands our tears. Amen.

The Journey

"The priest answered them, 'Go in peace. Your journey has the Lord's approval.'"

Judges 18:6 (NIV)

There is a story that dates to the early 1900s about a missionary who was traveling with a group of native porters across a portion of Africa. Anxious to reach his destination, he had been pushing the group hard for three days. On the morning of the fourth day, having himself eaten a hurried breakfast, the missionary prepared for another long day of traveling. He was taken back, however, when he discovered the porters leisurely relaxing over their breakfasts. The porters appeared as if they might well take all day to eat. The missionary ordered them to finish their breakfast and pack quickly so they could make the most of the daylight. Still, the porters refused to move. Stymied, the missionary asked the head porter to talk with the others in an attempt to determine the problem. After talking with his men, the head porter came back and told the missionary, "They said they're not going anywhere until their souls have time to catch up with their bodies."

1. Have you ever known anyone who has moved into a nursing home? Who?
   a. What were some of the things that person would liked to have taken but had to leave behind?
   b. What were some of the things that person considered important enough to bring along? Why do you think those things were so important?
2. If you had to move into a nursing home and could only take a few of your most prized possessions, what would

you take? Why are those particular items important to you?

3. Matthew 10:5-10 tells of Jesus sending his disciples out to work among the people. As you read these verses, consider:
   a. Why do you think they went out with few possessions?
   b. What do possessions tend to do to us?
   c. How would you simplify your life if you could?
   d. What is stopping you from taking action to simplify your life?

4. What have been some of the most precious things and who have been some of the most valued people you have had to let go of as you moved through your life? Give examples.

5. In the story, *Joseph,* we read about rest stops.
   a. What does it mean to rest: emotionally? physically? mentally? spiritually?
   b. What or who are your rest stops in life? Explain.

6. As you continue your journey, what *things* do you see in your covered wagon (see *Gilbert*) as being unnecessary?

7. If you were to die today, are there grudges you would carry to your grave? If you do not wish to carry them to your grave, what would you like to do about them?

8. Why do you think it is important to seek reconciliation as you journey through life? Discuss.

9. Wilma said she needed music to help her soul breathe. What do you think she meant by that? What kind of music would help your soul to breathe? Why that kind of music?

10. Reflect upon what the following verses might mean to you as you continue your journey:
    a. Psalm 25:4
    b. Proverbs 3:6
    c. Psalm 16:11
    d. John 4:6

Prayer
We ask for guidance as we continue on the journeys we are traveling. Remind us that we do not journey alone. Amen.

16

Saying Good-bye

"But when our time was up, we left and continued on our way. All the disciples and their wives and children accompanied us out of the city, and there on the beach we knelt to pray. After saying good-bye to each other, we went aboard the ship, and they returned home."

Acts 21:5 (NIV)

Life is a series of beginnings and endings, of hellos and good-byes. The good-byes are never easy. The only way to live life without experiencing the pain of separation when someone dies is to go through life without investing your love in others. While not loving others may be an option, it is certainly not a very appealing one, and I think it would leave you feeling empty inside. God has given us another option, though, and that is to love others. To invest our love in others, however, also means to feel the pain when they die. That is the risk we take when we love.

1. Have you ever been involved in the dying experience with someone for whom you have had special feelings? What were the circumstances?
    a. What was difficult for you?
    b. Were there blessings that came from the experience? If so, give details.
2. Have you ever been in a situation where you thought you might die? What were the circumstances?
    a. Looking back upon that experience, what goes through your mind now?
    b. In what ways, if any, has that experience changed your life? How has it affected your faith?
    c. What would be a *good death* for you?

3. In the story, *John,* the chaplain said that one's relationship is not to be measured in those last few moments before death. What do you think he meant?
4. Reflect upon the following statement: After your parents die, you become an orphan.
5. Regarding the story, *Betty:*
   a. Do you agree with her right to make the decision she did?
   b. What would you say to those who would see her decision as a form of suicide?
   c. Would you have made the same decision if you were her? Why or why not?
   d. How would your faith community view her decision?
   e. Would you see her decision as a quality of life, dignity, or a ethical issue? Explain.
6. If you were to die this day, what would be your greatest regret about life?
   a. For what in your life would you be most grateful?
   b. What would be the last thing you would want to do or say?
7. Some families have a short service at the bedside of the dying before or after death. They may read scripture, sing hymns, have prayers, etc. If you were to do hold a bedside service for your loved one—
   a. What hymns or songs would you select?
   b. What readings (sacred or secular) would you have?
   c. What would be your closing prayer or expression of thoughts?
8. Reflect upon the meaning of the following verses in light of Bess' story:
   a. Genesis 27:1-2
   b. Ecclesiastes 3:1-2
   c. I Corinthians 15:54-57
   d. Psalm 89:48

Prayer

Grant us patience as we approach the end of our journeys. Comfort us with the certain knowledge that we shall be taken home according to your will and timetable. Amen.

17

Going Home

"In my Father's house are many rooms; if it were not so, I would have told you. I am going there to prepare a place for you."

John 14:2 (NIV)

"Going home" is an expression that many residents use; it is symbolic language used in reference to their pending death. The truth is that while the thought of separation can be painful for the family, the thought of their loved one "going home" brings a certain amount of comfort and peace.

Our reactions toward death are often shaped by our initial experiences with it. In order to begin to understand why we deal with death the way we do, we need to reflect upon our early experiences and how they have shaped us in positive or negative ways.

1. What was the first death experience you recall? What were the circumstances?
    a. What were the feelings you remember having at that time?
    b. What do you remember regarding how the adults handled the death?
2. What "messages" were you given at the time? For example, little boys used to be told, "Don't cry. Be a man."
3. Have you ever had the experience of talking about death with someone who was terminally ill?
    a. Who? Describe the circumstances.
    b. Did that experience change you? If so, in what way?
4. Have you ever attended a funeral visitation where you have noticed one group of people smiling and laughing in one corner while in another corner of the room, people were crying?

a. If so, how would you explain that to a young person who is attending his or her first funeral visitation?

b. Do you recall your own first experience involving those circumstances? If so, share.

5. Thinking back to the last funeral you attended, what do you remember— Seeing? Hearing? Smelling? What emotions (feelings) did you have?

6. Have you planned or thought about your funeral? If so, share your thoughts. If you haven't, why not?

7. Read I Thessalonians 4:13 and John 11:35. On the surface, these two verses seem to contradict one another in terms of grieving.

   a. Can a person experience grief and still have a strong faith? Discuss.

   b. If you saw Jesus weeping, in what way would you comfort him?

8. The story entitled *Emma* uses the image of a pile of wheelchairs, walkers, etc. outside the gates of heaven. What will you leave on that pile as you walk through the gates?

9. The story, *Ebert*, talks about a booth in heaven where God will answer questions. What questions would you like to ask God at that booth? How do you think God will answer them?

10. What kind of questions do you have at the present time concerning life after death?

    a. How do you now address these questions? Are you satisfied with your answers? Why or why not?

    b. How do you think your faith community would address your questions?

11. Jesus talked about the Kingdom of God as a house with many rooms. Reflect upon the positive attributes of thinking of Heaven in that way.

12. How does Revelation 21:1-4 portray heaven?

Prayer

We praise your name for the lives of all our friends and loved ones who have *gone home*. We name them in our hearts as we pay honor to their memory (you may, if you so wish, say their names aloud). We give thanks for all they meant to us and how they touched our lives. Amen.

18

Angels

"Do not forget to entertain strangers, for by so doing some people have entertained angels without knowing it."

Hebrews 13:2 (NIV)

One of the roles of angels in Scripture was to bring God's Word into everyday life situations. They could announce some great event or proclaim a message of hope or provide a word of warning. They were seen as messengers of God, and their messages often were the catalysts for dramatic changes within the lives of people.

Modern-day angels come in all different sizes, colors and ages. They may not be wearing halos nor have wings, but nevertheless, they are here within our lives and they may leave their calling cards when we least expect it.

1. What kind of angels (pictures, statues, pins, books, etc.) do you have around your home? Why are these items meaningful to you?
2. When someone calls another an "angel," what is usually meant by that?
3. Do you think you have ever entertained angels without knowing it?
   a. What were the circumstances?
   b. Did they bring any "messages" (spiritual insights, wisdom, etc.) from God? Was your life changed in any way? Share, if you feel comfortable doing so.
4. Do you believe in guardian angels? Explain. Have there been occasions in your life when you have felt you had been watched over by an angel? If so, share.
5. What would you ask your guardian angel to protect you from today? Explain.

6. Angels are also there to give guidance. Are there areas in your life where guidance is needed? If you feel comfortable, share.
7. In the story, *Jacob*, there is reference to residents who saw angels before they died. Do you believe in such occurrences? Why or why not?
8. Have you ever known any "elderly angels?" Who were they? What message did they bring to you about life?
9. What do the following scripture passages tell you about angels:
   a. Hebrews 1:14
   b. Daniel 6:22
   c. Revelation 12:7-9
   d. Matthew 18:10
   e. I Kings 19:1-8
   f. Acts 12:7
10. II Corinthians 11:14 talks about how Satan can disguise himself as an angel of light. What do you think is meant by that? Have you ever had an experience with such an angel? If so, describe.
11. In the story, *Six Words*, the card that was left in the chaplain's office expressed three thoughts. How would you apply the following to spiritual growth and faith: Live Well. Laugh Often. Love Much.
    a. Have you known nursing home residents who did apply those words to their lives? Who were they and in what ways did they apply the words?
    b. What did you learn from those who did apply the words to their lives?
12. If you printed your philosophy of life on a business card, what would your card say?
13. If you were to design a business card for the angels of God, what would you put on it?

Prayer
Help us to discern the presence of angels and the messages they bring into our lives. We ask that our hearts might be opened to the expectation that we may be entertaining angels unaware the next time we visit residents who live in long term care facilities. Amen.

Order Form

Please Send Me:

_____ copies of *Study Guide* @ $4.95 per copy _____

_____ copies of *Seeing Beyond the Wrinkles* _____
    @ $12.95 per copy

California residents add 8.25% tax _____

Postage & handling for one item _____$2.50_____

Postage & handling for additional _____
    items @ 75¢ each

TOTAL ENCLOSED _____

Payment Type

❒ Check   ❒ Money Order   ❒ Visa

❒ Mastercard   ❒ Discover   ❒ American Express

Credit Card #:_____ Exp. Date:_____

Name:_____

Address:_____

City:_____ State:_____ Zip:_____

Make checks payable to: **Studio 4 Productions**
                                     P.O. Box 280400
                              Northridge, CA 91328-0400
                                         U.S.A.